A Report on Animal Longevity
BY BARBARA FORD

WHY DOES A TURTLE LIVE LONGER THAN A DOG?

ILLUSTRATED WITH PHOTOGRAPHS

William Morrow and Company   New York   1980

Library of Congress Cataloging in Publication Data

Ford, Barbara.
   Why does a turtle live longer than a dog?

   Includes index.
   Summary: Examines the variation in life-spans of both domestic and wild animals, ranging from one day to more than a century. Discusses ways of estimating age and theories on why life-spans vary and what causes aging.
   1. Longevity—Juvenile literature. 2. Life (Biology)—Juvenile literature. 3. Death (Biology)—Juvenile literature. [1. Longevity. 2. Animals—Age. 3. Life (Biology)] I. Title.
QP85.F67   591.3′74   79-28159
ISBN 0-688-22229-3
ISBN 0-688-32229-8 lib. bdg.

Printed in the United States of America.
   1   2   3   4   5   6   7   8   9   10

By Barbara Ford and Ronald R. Keiper
THE ISLAND PONIES
An Environmental Study of Their Life on Assateague

ACKNOWLEDGMENTS

Many people and organizations helped make this book possible. My special thanks to the following, listed in alphabetical order:

Dion A. Albach, Mesker Park Zoo
Dr. Wilbur B. Amand, J. Kevin Bowler, Philadelphia Zoo
William A. Austin, Detroit Zoo
Frank A. Bailey, National Marine Fisheries Service
John Beecham, Idaho Department of Fish and Game
Bea Boone, Gary L. Krapu, United States Fish and Wildlife Service
Charles River Breeding Laboratories
Gary K. Clarke, Topeka Zoo
Dr. Bennett J. Cohen, Professor Richard W. Dapson,
    University of Michigan
Dr. Lanny H. Cornell, Sea World
Dover Pet Shop
Mr. and Mrs. Fred Falkenbach
Clayton F. Freiheit, Denver Zoo
Renate Graf, Lion Country Safari
Dr. David E. Harrison, The Jackson Laboratory
Dr. George Y. Harry, Jr., National Marine Mammal Laboratory
Dr. Ronald W. Hart, Ohio State University
James Hunsinger, Turtleback Zoo
King Ranch, Inc.
Bob Kuhn, Oregon Department of Fish and Wildlife
Robert C. Lund, New Jersey Department of Environmental Protection
Tim Morefield, Dave Ramczyk, and Tom Taylor,
    California Department of Fish and Game
New Zealand Consulate General
Mrs. Alice Newman
Dr. Svend W. Nielsen, University of Connecticut
Oregon Historical Society
Parrot Jungle
Dr. George B. Rabb, Brookfield Zoo
Ann Redelfs, Oklahoma City Zoo
Jimmy R. Roberts, Yerkes Regional Primate Research Center
Professor Morris Rockstein, University of Miami School of Medicine
Mark A. Rosenthal, Lincoln Park Zoo
Mr. and Mrs. Fred Stevenson
Bob Truett, Birmingham Zoo
Mrs. Mildred Wein, Noah's Ark Shelter
Charles G. Wilson, Memphis Zoo
William L. Wilson, New Jersey Marine Sciences Consortium

For Frank Kendig

CONTENTS

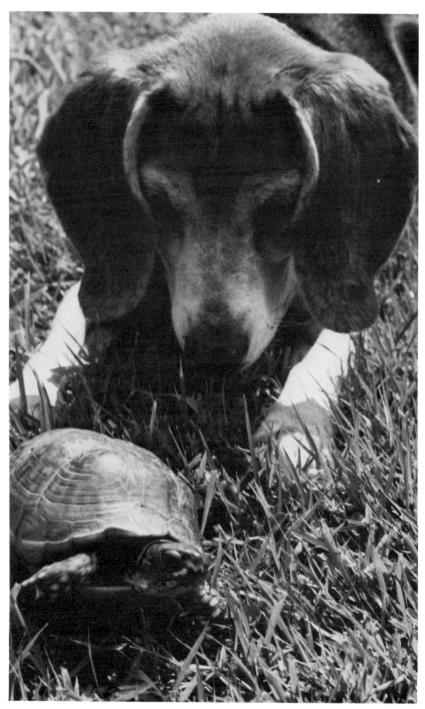

THE LIFE-SPAN
OF TAME ANIMALS

My beagle dog, Luci, had her twelfth birthday this year. She is in good health, but at twelve she is an old dog. Most medium-sized dogs like beagles live only fourteen to fifteen years. I don't know how old my eastern box turtle, Beebs, is, but she was already an adult when she was captured five years ago. Yet Beebs will probably outlive my dog; in fact, a few box turtles are known to have lived over a century. My toads, Greenie and Brownie, will probably outlive Luci too; some toads reach their thirties.

The only pets I have that probably won't outlive Luci are my anole lizards, Ann and Noel, who are two to three years old. Anoles live a maximum of four years in captivity, making them one of the shortest-lived reptiles.

As these ages show, animal life-spans—the average age animals of a species can expect to reach—vary enormously. So do their maximum longevities, the oldest age reached by an individual in a species. These wide variations are found throughout the animal kingdom, but we notice them more among pets and domesticated animals. After all, they are under our observation.

What do records tell us about the ages of creatures closest to us, like pets and farm animals?

The eastern box turtle, which many people keep as a pet, lives longer than any other animal associated with man. Two individuals of this small species of turtle are known to have lived 123 and 129 years. The 129-year record was set by a turtle that was marked and released early in the 1800's, then recaptured more than a century later. Some other turtles found in this country are fairly long-lived, but most are not suitable as pets. An exception is the diamondback terrapin, a medium-sized water turtle also popular as food. One lived for forty years in captivity, and people who have kept them say they make good pets.

Turtles are reptiles, a group of cold-blooded animals. They and their relatives, the amphibians, include many long-lived creatures. Some are popular for the home terrarium. The slow worm, which is really a lizard, is a reptile that does well in captivity and is also long-lived. One survived fifty-four years in captivity. The glass snake, which is a relative of the slow worm and a lizard also, can live up to twenty-five years. It flourishes in captivity too. Another lizard that has reached a quarter century is the iguana. Many of these large, green lizards (they grow to six feet if given large quarters) are sold in pet shops today. The true toad, an amphibian and a close relative of the common toads of the United States, has lived thirty-six years in captivity.

All the long-lived snakes are big, so more suitable for zoos than most homes. An example is the boa. The oldest snake known is a South African boa, which was forty in 1979. It lives in the Philadelphia Zoo. Boas become quite docile in captivity according to snake experts.

Some birds kept as pets live as long as all but the longest-lived turtles. A greater sulphur-crested cockatoo, the most popular of the cockatoos, lived to the age of fifty-six in captivity. An individual of this species spent forty years entertaining the public at Parrot Jungle in Miami, Florida. Cockatoos in general are long-lived birds, half a dozen species reaching their thirties or forties. An African gray parrot, the best talker of the parrots, has reached fifty. Other records set by birds kept as pets are a blue-and-yellow macaw, forty-three; a domestic pigeon, thirty; and an Indian Hill mynah, twenty. All these birds are big, but one canary lived to twenty-two and a budgie, a small parakeet, to fifteen.

Among the longer-lived pets is the goldfish. There are records of a few goldfish reaching thirty and even forty years of age, although the average life-span is about seventeen.

Our most popular pets, the dog and cat, are short-lived compared to many birds and reptiles. Medium-sized and small dogs usually live about fifteen years, large dogs a year or two less. The oldest dog known died at twenty-seven. He was Adjutant, a Labrador retriever, who lived on a country estate in England from 1936 to 1963.

Dog experts no longer believe that one year in the life of a dog is equal to seven in the life of a human being. The current thinking is that at one year a dog's development is like that of a sixteen-year-old person. At two, the dog is like a twenty-four-year-old, at three, it is like a thirty-year-old, and at four, it is comparable to a thirty-five-year-old. After four, each year in a dog's life is equivalent to five in a human being's life. Using this formula, Adjutant would have been 150 in human terms.

Cats normally live a year or two longer than dogs. There are records of two cats reaching thirty-one, one a male and one a female. Surveys of cat owners in the United States, Britain, and Canada have turned up a number of cats over twenty.

Among the animals we domesticate for agriculture and other purposes, horses live the longest. There is a good record for one mare living forty-six years, and several records for horses over forty. Arabian horses are noted for their longevity, and records of thoroughbred horses show a small number of Arabians, most of them mares, have lived into their thirties. Famous

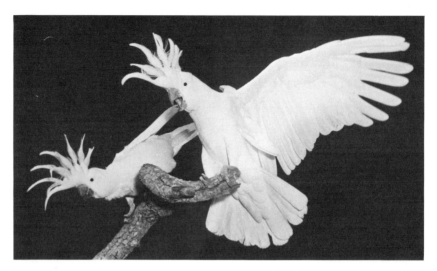

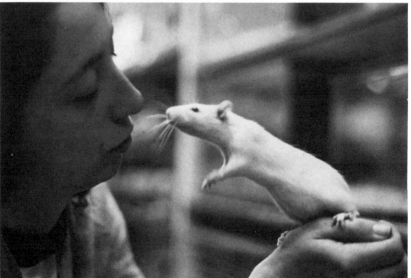

Top: Butch, the greater sulphur-crested cockatoo on the right, lived into his forties at Parrot Jungle in Miami, Florida. He once sat on the shoulder of Winston Churchill. *Parrot Jungle*

Bottom: Small rodents are among the shortest-lived pets. White rats such as this one at the Dover Pet Shop, Dover, New Jersey, live no more than six years. *Barbara Ford*

Opposite: Marthur, a female Maine coon cat, caught a mouse in 1979, when she was nineteen years old. She belongs to Mrs. Alice Newman of Boonton Township, New Jersey. *Barbara Ford*

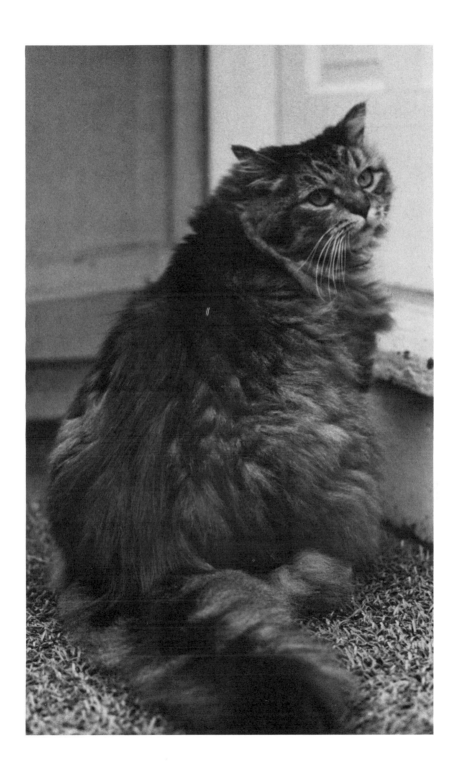

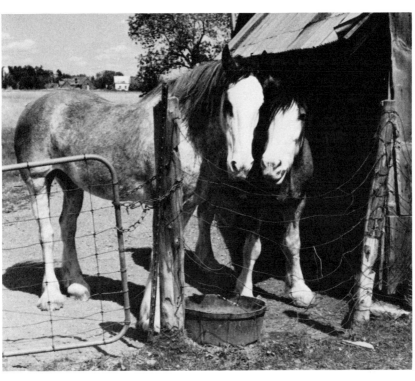

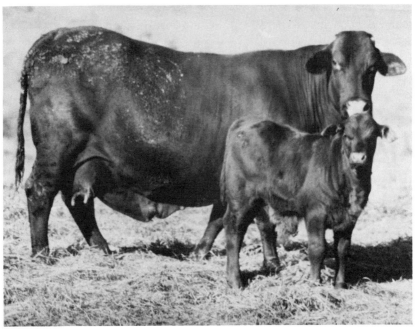

racehorses are often retired at an early age and allowed to live out their lives. Some of them reach advanced ages. Man O'War, one of the most renowned racehorses, reached the age of thirty. He was buried in a satin-lined coffin in Lexington, Kentucky.

The cow has a maximum age of about thirty, but few live even half that long. Most cows, like other farm animals, are killed for meat or because they are not productive. Still, a few cows do live fairly long lives. On the famous King Ranch in Texas, one of the largest ranches in the world, there is a herd of Santa Gertrudis cattle, a breed noted for its longevity. One cow in this herd was twenty-three in 1979 and had just had her twentieth calf. Most cows do well to bear ten calves.

Both the sheep and the hog have a maximum longevity of about twenty years. Oddly enough, the little domestic rabbit has a maximum almost as long, and some rabbits are still breeding at eighteen. The chicken lives ten years at best.

Some animals kept as pets have unusually short lives, particularly small rodents. The maximum age for a guinea pig is eight years, for a hamster about half that long, for a white rat about six years, and for a white mouse two to three years. One gerbil lived in the London Zoo for over five years, which was a record. Garter snakes do a little better than small rodents, one having reached the age of ten in captivity. The shortest-lived pet is probably the tiny goby fish, a popular aquarium species, which lives only about a year.

Top: After fifteen years of pulling wagonloads of tourists through an experimental farm in Canada, these two Clydesdale horses retired. Both are twenty-three, an old age for this big, stocky breed of horse.
Agriculture Canada
Bottom: At twenty-three, this Santa Gertrudis cow had her twentieth calf.
King Ranch, Inc.

THE LIFE-SPAN
OF WILD ANIMALS

The clams you eat in your chowder may be some of the oldest animals in the world. New Jersey scientists recently discovered, off the coast of New Jersey, quahog clams that are 149 years old. The ancient clams showed no signs of age, and they may be capable of living even longer. The quahog is the oldest clam known, but there is a European freshwater clam that is believed to live over a century.

Clams are invertebrates, members of a very large group of animals that lack a spinal column, or backbone. The invertebrates include not only some of the longest-lived animals, but all of the shortest-lived creatures.

Besides the clam, the longest-lived invertebrate known is the sea anemone, a simple, flowerlike animal that lives on the bottom of the ocean. One colony of sea anemones was put in an aquarium in the Department of Zoology at the University of Edinburgh, Scotland, sometime before 1862. In 1942, they died from unknown causes.

During their long life in the aquarium the anemones showed no signs of age, so they, too, may be capable of living to greater ages than those recorded. In fact, animals like the sea anemone and clam may not grow old at all. They may simply go on living until an accident ends their life.

No other invertebrates are known to live quite as long as sea anemones and clams, but some survive for a surprisingly long time. Certain mussels, relatives of the clam, may live a half century or more. The age of the American lobster cannot be determined precisely, but it may also live a half century. The big, hairy tarantula spider can live up to a quarter century, and so can the queen termite, an insect. The tapeworm, a parasitic worm that lives in the human body, may have a life-span of up to thirty-five years—within the body of its human host. The noisy seventeen-year cicada, familiar to us as a flying insect, spends most of its seventeen-year life-span underground in a crawling form called a "nymph."

Some invertebrates measure their life in days, not years. The shortest-lived animal of all is the mayfly, an insect that lives only a day or so as an adult. Another very short-lived invertebrate is the housefly, which lives seventeen to twenty-nine days on the average. The longest-lived houseflies reach two months.

In between the extremes are invertebrates with life-spans of months and years. The angular-winged katydid, the bright-green insect familiar in our backyards in summer, lives about five months. The American cockroach, biggest of the cockroaches at two inches, lives six to seven months. Worker bees can live up to six years. Worker ants can live four to seven years, their queen up to fifteen years. Some medium-sized spiders have been kept alive in captivity up to nine years. The earthworm can live six years.

The rest of the animal world is made up of vertebrates, animals with a spinal column. Vertebrates are divided into four large groups: reptiles and amphibians, fish, birds, and mammals. Each group has its long- and short-lived members.

To the reptiles and amphibians belongs what is believed to be the oldest animal that ever lived. In 1766, French explorer Marion de Fresne captured an adult giant tortoise in the Seychelles Islands in the Indian Ocean and took it to another Indian Ocean island, Mauritius. There it lived in an

15

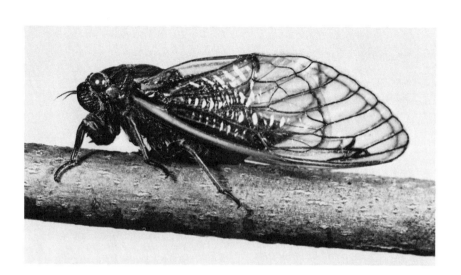

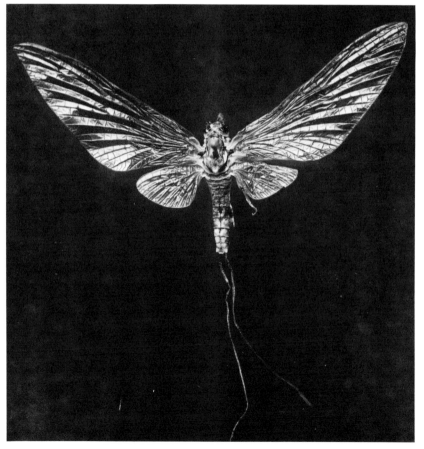

Army barracks in the town of Fort Louis until it tumbled into a hole in 1918 and died of its injuries. It had lived in captivity 152 years, but as it was an adult when captured, it must have been older. The giant Seychelles tortoise has been exterminated on its native island, but survives on another nearby.

Another giant tortoise, the huge Galápagos seen in zoos, has lived over 100 years in captivity.

Next to the turtles, the longest-lived reptile is the tuatara, a strange, lizardlike creature about two feet long that is found only in New Zealand. One lived seventy-seven years in captivity. A number of reptiles reach their fifties or sixties in captivity, including North American species such as the snapping turtle and musk turtle. The Philadelphia Zoo has two ancient alligator snapping turtles, one of which was sixty-two and the other fifty-eight in 1979. Other fifty-year-plus reptiles or amphibians are the American alligator, whose record is fifty-six, and the Japanese giant salamander, whose record is fifty-five. The latter, a native of Japan and China, is now rare. It sometimes grows to almost six feet in length.

The longest-lived fish known is the sturgeon. In 1951, a sturgeon caught in the northwestern United States was found to be eighty-two years old. It weighed 900 pounds, was 11½ feet long, and gave between 150 and 200 pounds of caviar. Caviar is a name for sturgeon eggs, which are much prized by people who enjoy unusual food. A sturgeon caught in Russia that weighed 2200 pounds and was 13 feet long was said by scientists to be seventy-five years old.

Sturgeon may grow throughout life, or at least well past the age of maturity (the age at which animals can mate and bear

---

Top: The seventeen-year cicada exists only a few weeks as a winged insect after spending most of its life underground.
United States Department of Agriculture

Bottom: The delicate mayfly has the shortest life of any animal—one day.
United States Department of Agriculture

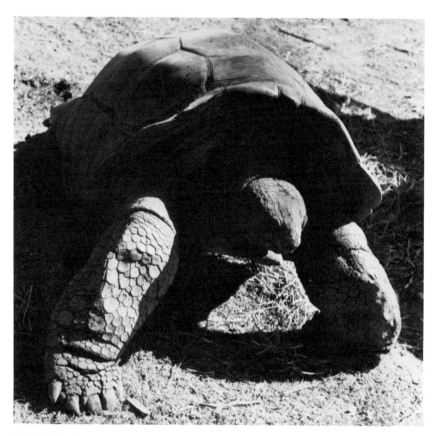

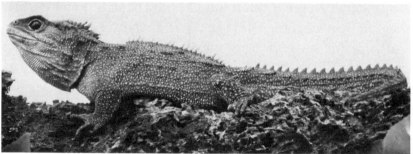

Top: This sturdy Aldabra tortoise is an estimated sixty to seventy years old, but it may see the year 2000.

George Walters, Oklahoma City Zoo, Oklahoma

Bottom: One New Zealand tuatara lived seventy-seven years in captivity.

New Zealand Consulate General, New York

Opposite: This eighty-two-year-old sturgeon is the oldest fish known.

Oregon Historical Society

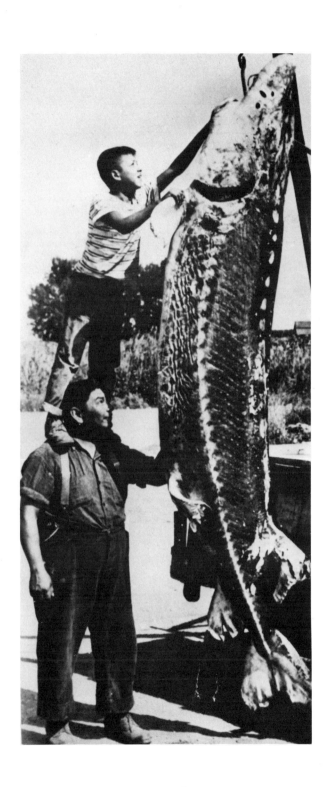

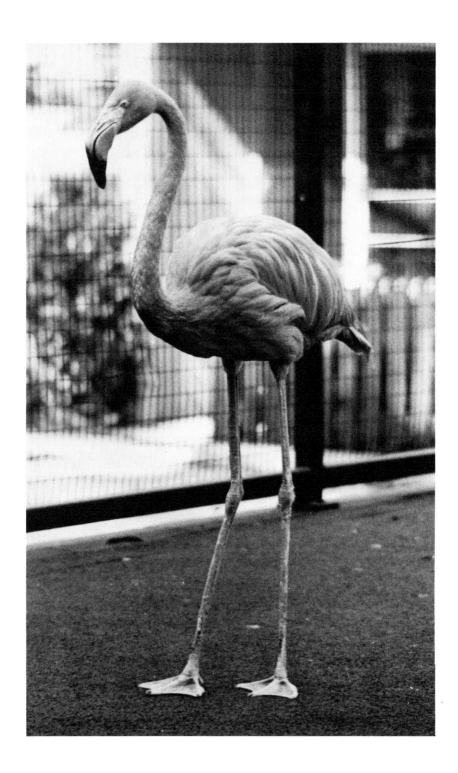

young). This same growth pattern is found among some other big fish as well as certain reptiles.

Once it was believed that as long as a fish or reptile kept growing, it would not age, but this theory has been disproved. Some fish die of old age while still growing.

Regardless, long-lived fish, most of them big species, are not uncommon. The halibut and European catfish have both reached the age of sixty, and several eels have lived into their fifties. At Shedd Aquarium in Chicago, there were five fish in their forties in 1979: two sturgeon, two Australian lungfish, and a tarpon, a game fish, which was eight feet long. Some carp also reach forty in aquariums. Two sharks, the spiny dogfish and the Australian school shark, are known to have lived at least thirty years in the wild. The dogfish and longnose gar, both North American freshwater species, have reached thirty in aquariums.

While no birds have an extremely long maximum age none have an extremely short life either. The oldest bird known was a sixty-eight-year-old eagle owl, a European relative of our great horned owl and the biggest owl in Europe (twenty-six inches). Other wild birds with a long maximum age are the Andean condor, sixty-five years; the Asiatic crane, sixty; the bateleur eagle, fifty-five; the vasa parrot, fifty-four; the golden-naped parrot, forty-nine; the Australian crane, forty-seven; the golden eagle, forty-six; the herring gull, forty-one; the king vulture, forty; the American crane, thirty-eight; the California condor, thirty-seven, and the emperor penguin, thirty-four. All are sizable birds, for among birds, as among fish, large size often goes with long life.

The oldest known age of a small bird is the thirty-year record set by a red-crested cardinal. An English sparrow reached

---

Among birds, large size often goes with long life. This greater flamingo is twenty years old. *Birmingham Zoo, Alabama*

twenty-three, a starling seventeen, and both a purple grackle and a blue jay lived to fourteen.

The life-spans of mammals probably interest us more than those of any other animal because we ourselves are mammals. The human species is by far the longest-lived of them all. According to the *Guinness Book of World Records*, the oldest human being for whom there are good records was a New York State resident, Mrs. Delina Filkins, who died at 113. The maximum age of our closest animal relatives, the great apes, is only half as long as ours. One orangutan lived to the age of fifty-nine in a zoo. The oldest gorilla, Massa, who lives in the Philadelphia Zoo, and the oldest chimpanzee, Bula, at Yerkes Regional Primate Center, Atlanta, Georgia, are both forty-nine. There are several records of forty-seven-year-old chimps.

At least one species of monkey lives as long as apes. Bobo, a capuchin at Mesker Park Zoo in Evansville, Indiana, is believed to be forty-nine. His capuchin companion, Jerry, died at the zoo in 1976 at the age of forty-seven. A few other monkeys reach their thirties.

The longest-lived mammal next to the human being is the Indian elephant. One died in an Australian zoo at an age estimated to be sixty-nine to seventy-seven, after living at the zoo fifty-seven years. Victor B. Scheffer, an American biologist who is an expert on marine mammals, believes some sperm whales also live into their seventies. He bases this estimate on sperm whale teeth. In his book, *A Natural History of Marine Mammals*, Scheffer points out that a male killer whale with peculiar markings was sighted along the Australian coast for more than ninety years. Two other whales, the finback and the pilot, are believed to reach the age of fifty years.

No other mammal is known to live as long as whales and elephants, but a small number reach their forties and even fifty. A spiny anteater lived in captivity for forty-nine years. There is a record of forty-six years for a gray seal and forty for an African black rhinoceros. According to a study made in Rwenzori National Park in Uganda, Africa, most wild hippopotamuses live into their forties in a protected situation. Unfortunately, many of the hippos in this park were killed in 1979 by invading Tanzanian soldiers. The wild walrus is also believed to reach forty.

In 1974, a wild black bear shot in New York State by hunters was found to be forty-one years old, a record for bears of any species. Individuals among all of the big bears, as well as the lion, the zebra, the camel, the fruit bat, and the genet (a small spotted animal that looks like a cat), are known to have passed their thirtieth birthday in captivity.

Almost all other mammals have much shorter lives, including those most familiar to us. A gray squirrel and a badger have a maximum age of twenty-three, a raccoon twenty-two, a white-tailed deer twenty, a red fox twelve, a North American porcupine ten, a striped skunk ten, a cottontail rabbit nine, a chipmunk eight, and a house mouse three. All these ages were set in captivity. The shortest-lived mammal, and one of the shortest-lived vertebrates, is the tiny shrew. It lives only a little over a year at best.

Overleaf, top left: Bertie, a twenty-three-year-old male hippo, is middle-aged by hippo standards.   *Denver Zoological Gardens, Colorado*
Bottom left: Mike, the big polar bear on the left, was at least thirty-two when he died.   *Lincoln Park Zoological Garden, Chicago, Illinois*
Top right: Frasier was an estimated seventeen to twenty years old when he came to Lion Country Safari, but he soon acquired a harem of seven lionesses and sired thirty-three cubs. He died in 1972.
Lion Country Safari, California
Bottom right: This female American elk is over twenty years of age, making her one of the oldest elks in captivity. She has had six offspring and they have had three more. Her keeper calls her Granny Goat.
Birmingham Zoo, Alabama

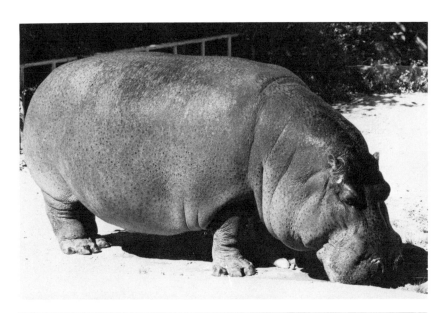

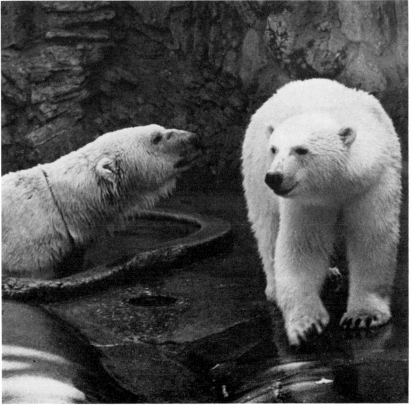

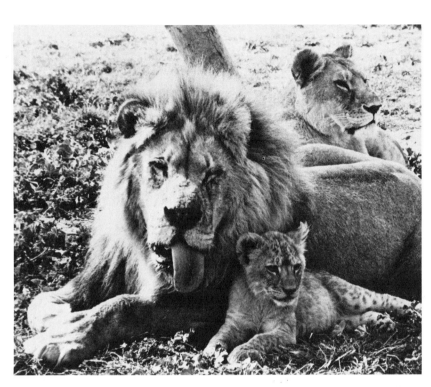

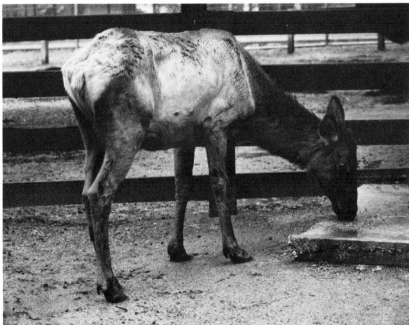

TELLING AGE

Telling the age of a domesticated animal or a wild animal in captivity is easy as these creatures have been under our observation since they were born or captured. Telling the age of animals in the wild is much harder. We usually can distinguish very young animals by size and other characteristics, but after maturity the age of many wild animals is difficult to judge. There are methods for doing so, however. These methods were developed by scientists who needed age data to help them make decisions about how to manage animals in the wild.

State government biologists, for instance, need information about the age of game animals to establish hunting regulations. If statistics show that not enough animals of a species reach the age where they can mate and have young, the biologists may shorten the hunting season or even suspend it.

The same kind of data is used by scientists responsible for nongame animals and animals in protected areas like parks.

Top: Two ear tags were placed on this four-year-old black bear in Idaho as part of a population study. Bears often lose tags.
John Beecham, Idaho Department of Fish and Game
Bottom: A Canada goose is banded.
Luther C. Goldman, United States Fish and Wildlife Service

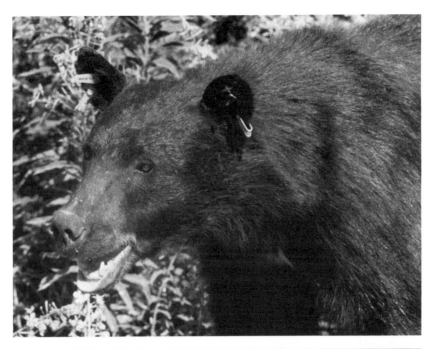

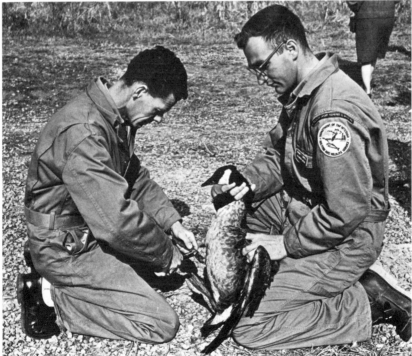

One way scientists get data is by tagging animals. That is, they capture the animal, put some kind of marker on it, and then release it. If it is captured again, there is a record of how long the animal has been in the wild. Some of the maximum age records come from tagged animals, including the 129-year-old box turtle, thirty-two-year-old Australian school shark, and a twenty-four-year-old bighorn sheep. Probably more birds are tagged than any other animal. Among birds, the practice usually is known as banding because a metal band is put around the bird's leg. The oldest banded bird known was a European oyster catcher, which had been tagged thirty-two years before it was recaptured.

Tagging supplies valuable information, but tagged animals are not always recovered and many species cannot be tagged. So scientists use additional ways to determine age.

For many big mammals, teeth are a good indicator of age. There are two methods of telling an animal's age by its teeth. One is called the "eruption-and-wear-pattern method." Among many species, including human beings, young animals have baby teeth that fall out as the animal matures. They are replaced by adult teeth that appear, or erupt, at certain times. By checking which baby teeth are present and how many adult teeth have erupted, an expert can tell the age of an animal that does not yet have all its adult teeth.

The wear pattern gives even more information. The teeth of a young white-tailed deer, for instance, are high and sharp. As it ages, the teeth become lower and rounder. Some of the teeth of a ten-year-old deer are worn almost to the gum line or even below it.

Putting these two kinds of information together, someone familiar with the eruption-and-wear-pattern method can tell the age of animals very quickly. Robert C. Lund, a biologist with the New Jersey Department of Environmental Protection, says an experienced biologist can determine the age of a white-tailed deer in seconds. Each year Lund and other New Jersey state biologists use the eruption-and-wear method to age about 7000 white-tailed deer killed by hunters in the state's two-week deer season. Other states with deer-hunting seasons use the same method to age deer.

Though the eruption-and-wear method is widely used, it is not as accurate as another tooth-based method, particularly for older animals. This second method is called the "cementum-annuli technique." Cementum is the substance around the root of the tooth that holds it to the jawbone. *Annuli* is a Greek word for ring. If you look at a specially prepared section of tooth cementum under a microscope, you can see rings in it. Each ring corresponds to a year in the animal's life. When this technique is used on white-tailed deer, researchers usually choose an incisor, or front tooth, in the lower jaw for examination.

The cementum-annuli method works with a wide variety of mammals, including elk, pronghorn antelope, moose, bighorn sheep, bison, black bear, grizzly bear, raccoons, and coyotes. Beside accuracy, another advantage to this method is that it can be used on live wild animals as well as on dead ones. In many states, biologists are now trapping black bears, extracting a single tooth, and then releasing the animal. The tooth pulled is a premolar, a small tooth at the side of the jaw. Its loss does not bother the bear. One of the areas where live black bears are being aged this way is the Great Smoky Mountains National Park in Tennessee and North Carolina. The oldest bear found there was a fifteen-year-old female. Live coyotes and badgers in Idaho are also being aged with the cementum-annuli technique.

In addition, teeth reveal the age of some marine mammals such as whales and the fur seals that live on our Pribilof Islands off Alaska. In the case of fur seals, you can see ridges on the outside of the canine teeth, the long, pointed teeth at the corners of the jaw. Each ridge represents one year of life. Two scientists at the United States Department of Commerce's Na-

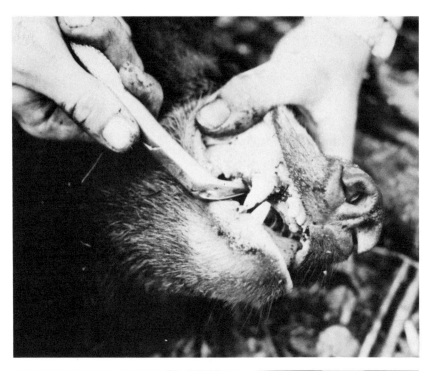

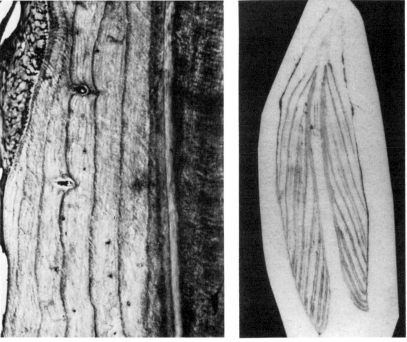

tional Marine Mammal Laboratory in Seattle, Washington, recently developed a way to make these ridges easier to read. In seals, unlike land mammals, what is read is the tooth dentine, the material that makes up most of the tooth.

While studying teeth is the best way to tell the ages of many large mammals, the method doesn't work very well with small mammals. To age these animals, scientists use another method: eye-lens weight. The eye lens increases in weight as the animal ages, and because it is not affected by the environment, it is a good indicator of age. After a certain age, however, the lens-weight method becomes inaccurate too. A better method based on the weight of the protein in the eye lens was developed recently by Professor Richard W. Dapson of the University of Michigan. The new method is based on the fact that lens protein changes in a certain way as an animal ages and the changes can be measured.

The Dapson method is now considered the most accurate way to age many small mammals. It can be used on other mammals, too, but since it requires special equipment it is not always practical.

Scientists have also worked out ways to age animals that have no teeth, like some fish and invertebrates. In the case of fish, age can often be read from growth rings on body structures such as scales and earplugs, or otoliths. Scales are the structures used most often, since removing a few of them does not harm the fish. Normally, the scale is pressed into heat-softened

---

Top: How do you pull a live bear's tooth? Carefully. This Maine black bear was tranquilized before biologists pulled a small premolar to determine its age. *Maine Department of Inland Fisheries and Wildlife*
Left: The cementum annuli on this white-tailed deer's tooth show it was six and one-half years old. The first ring in whitetails counts for a half year, as the young are born in May.
Joyce A. Czikowsky, Northwestern Research Center for Wildlife Diseases
Right: The age rings on a fur seal's tooth show it was nine years old.
National Oceanic and Atmospheric Association

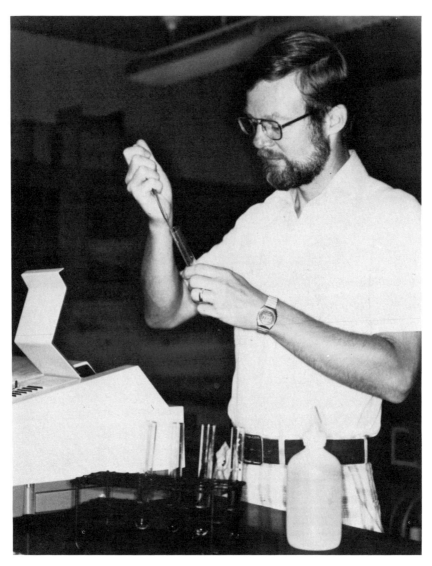

Richard W. Dapson measures protein content of eye lenses using a machine called a "spectrophotometer." *Paul Adams*

Opposite, top: The growth rings on this striped bass otolith indicate it was five years old. *Tom Taylor, California Department of Fish and Game*

Inset: These otoliths, shown actual size, come from a haddock.

National Marine Fisheries Service

Bottom: The growth rings of older fish are close together and hard to count. This cross section of a sturgeon fin ray shows it was twenty-one years old. *Tom Taylor, California Department of Fish and Game*

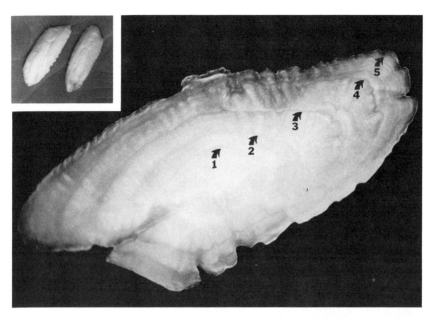

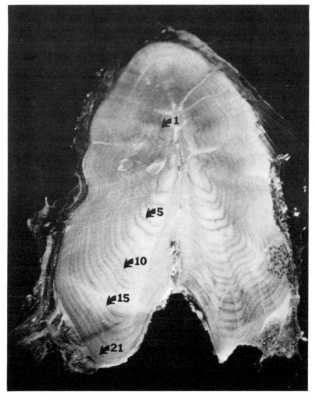

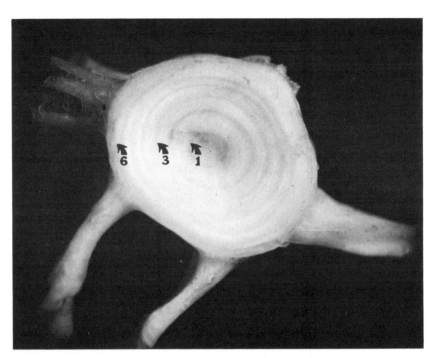

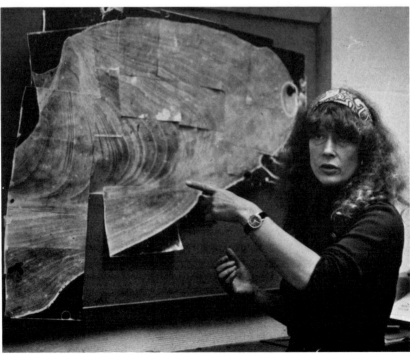

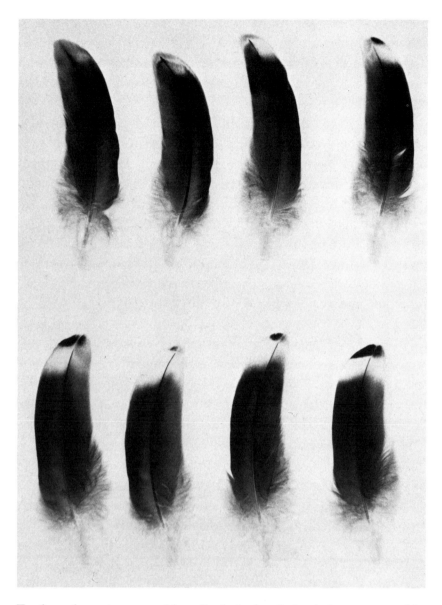

Feathers from two-year-old mallard ducks (below) have more white than feathers from year-old mallards (above).

United States Fish and Wildlife Service

Opposite, top: The spinal vertebra of this catfish has six growth rings, making it six years old. *Tom Taylor, California Department of Fish and Game*

Bottom: Ida Thompson points out age rings on this enlargement of the shell of a quahog clam. *New Jersey Marine Sciences Consortium*

plastic to make an impression, and then the impression is examined under a microscope. If a fish has no scales, the next best structures to read are otoliths, small, stonelike objects in the ear that are part of the fish's sensory and balancing mechanism.

If the fish has neither otoliths nor scales, spines, fin rays, and even bones can be read. The only reason we have an age record (thirty years) for the spiny dogfish is that its spines can be read under a microscope. Sharks have no true bones, no scales, no otoliths, and their teeth cannot be read.

Some clams have readable growth rings. The age of the 149-year-old clams found off New Jersey was determined by means of rings. Dr. Ida Thompson of Princeton University, the principal investigator in this project, developed a method by which the shells were sliced into thin peels that revealed the rings. The rings were then studied through a microscope or by means of enlarged photographs. As clams grow at different rates depending on their environment, scientists need to know the conditions under which they live in order to count their rings accurately. These conditions are known for the New Jersey clams, so their ages are probably correct.

One of the hardest animals to age is the bird. The eye-lens-protein method doesn't work with birds, and they have no teeth or other structures that might show growth rings. Birds do have feathers, however, and biologists who work with game birds have figured out how to age some game birds by using them. One bird they have studied is the mallard duck. Three members of the United States Fish and Wildlife Service's Northern Prairie Wildlife Research Center in Jamestown, North Dakota, have found that adult female mallards have a much larger area of white on some feathers than younger birds. Among young birds, these same feathers are mostly black.

The feather method doesn't give the exact age of the bird, but it does allow the biologists to figure out how many young and mature birds they have in a population.

WHY SOME ANIMALS
LIVE LONGER

We know how to age many animals in the wild, but most of the very old animals described in this book are pets or live in zoos or laboratories. In general, animals in protected situations live longer than the same animals in the wild. Scientists who study wild creatures tell us that the vast majority die from disease, accidents, hunting, or some other environmental cause before they ever reach their maximum age. One expert estimates that two-thirds of wild songbirds such as the robin and sparrow die in their first year. Bigger birds like the herring gull live only a little longer on the average.

Another expert found that the Indian mongoose, a small mammal, was old and almost toothless at three years of age in the wild. He could find no four-year-old mongooses. But in captivity the mongoose can live a dozen or more years. The record is seventeen.

Because most captive animals live longer, their ages are the ones that set the records. One of the first scientists to make a careful study of animal ages was the late Major Stanley S. Flower, a British naturalist. The Flower age lists are still in use. Major Flower refused to accept any records that did not have good evidence to back them up, and he depended heavily on zoo and kennel files as well as on carefully checked reports from pet owners. The same sources are used by modern scientists who collect animal age records today.

There are exceptions to the rule that animals live longer in protected surroundings. The age records for the sturgeon, the box turtle, the sperm whale, and the hippopotamus, among others, were achieved in the wild. Good health, a favorable environment, and luck probably determine which wild animals survive to be old. In 1960, a male bighorn lamb was released in Aravaipa Canyon, Arizona, by the Arizona Game and Fish Department. The lamb grew up to be a huge ram with a magnificent set of curled horns. He was often seen by visitors, but as hunting bighorns is not permitted in the canyon he was not harmed.

The ram wasn't sighted in 1976, and in December of that year his skeleton was found, complete with horns. They were a record size, forty-four and a half and forty-four inches. The Aravaipa ram did not establish an age record for bighorns (that was set by a twenty-four-year-old wild female), but he was among the oldest wild male bighorns.

But even under the best conditions there are still wide differences in animal ages. Why are laboratory mice old at two, while the average human being lives into his seventies? Why does the box turtle pass a century on this earth while the anole lizard seldom reaches its fourth birthday? Why is the life-span of the Mayfly a day, the honeybee six years, and the anemone an indefinite period of time?

There really are no complete answers to these questions,

Top: The Atlantic salmon lives longer than its Pacific cousins.
Luther C. Goldman, United States Fish and Wildlife Service
Bottom: Bottlenose dolphins mature late, carry their young in their bodies for many months, and bear one calf at a time, all factors linked with longevity. These lively old dolphins are estimated to be twenty-five to thirty. Maximum age in the wild is about thirty-five.
Sea World, San Diego, California

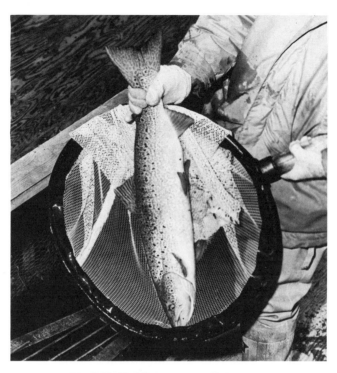

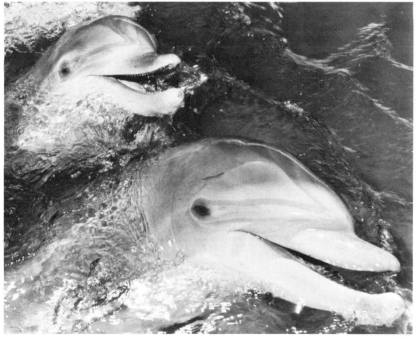

but there is old and new scientific research that sheds light on the subject.

One factor that affects life-span is reproduction. Scientists have known for many years that some animals die after reproducing once. Other creatures reproduce numerous times. Many insects and a few fish are in the first group, while most other animals fall into the second. Animals that reproduce once tend to have a short life-span, but they remain young for most of it. Animals that reproduce many times tend to have longer life-spans, but go through a period of old age.

The Pacific salmon is one well-known animal that belongs to the first group. Soon after laying its eggs for the first time, it dies. Its maximum age is about seven years, most of which it spends in an immature stage. The Atlantic salmon does not die after egg laying and has a maximum age of thirteen years.

The majority of the world's animals do not die after reproduction. In the case of many mammals, longevity is related to the age at which an animal becomes mature and the period of time it carries its young in its body before birth. The longer it takes an animal to develop and the longer it carries its young, the longer it lives. Human beings, the great apes, the brown bear, the whale, and the elephant all fit this pattern. These animals have small numbers of young, too. In a sense, these animals *have* to live a long time in order to replace themselves in the population.

New research reveals other information about animal ages. Dr. George A. Sacher of the United States Department of Energy's Argonne National Laboratory in Argonne, Illinois, has found four factors that seem to play a role in animal longevity. They are body size, brain size, metabolism (body processes that produce the energy the body needs), and body temperature. By means of complex mathematical formulas he has worked out, Dr. Sacher can show that these four factors account for most of the variation in animal life-spans.

The first factor of size is obvious. Most of the long-lived

animals are large. Elephants are huge, as are whales, hippopotamuses, and rhinoceroses, all of them among the longest-lived mammals. Horses, another long-lived mammal, are big too. Among the birds and fish, the bigger species live longer than the smaller ones. Big snakes and big turtles also live a long time.

There are many exceptions, though, such as the long-lived but small box turtle and the human being, who isn't a particularly large animal compared to many other mammals.

A better way to explain age, Sacher's formulas show, is brain size. In general, animals with big brains live longer than animals with small brains. The link between brain size and longevity is even more marked if brain size is considered apart from body size. The human species has a very large brain, and we live much longer than other mammals our size and even larger. The great apes, too, have large brains and live comparatively long lives. The elephant and whale are other large-brained, long-lived animals. A large brain is associated with intelligence as well as a long life, so intelligence may have something to do with life-span too.

Metabolism helps explain other puzzling age data. Have you ever watched a white mouse go through its daily activities? It moves so quickly that its tiny body fairly trembles. White mice and other very small warm-blooded mammals like the rat and shrew have high metabolism, which means their body has to

---

Overleaf, left: This photograph of Ziggy, one of the oldest and largest male elephants known, was taken when he was fifty-three. He died at age fifty-five. Elephants grow six sets of teeth, each of which lasts up to ten years. When the last set is gone, the elephant cannot eat normally; their maximum age is around seventy. *Brookfield Zoo, Illinois*
Top right: Large size is often linked with longevity. Horses, much bigger than dogs, live twice as long. *Barbara Ford*
Bottom right: Most snakes that reach old age are big ones. This king cobra was an adult when it first went on display in 1960.
Detroit Zoo, Michigan

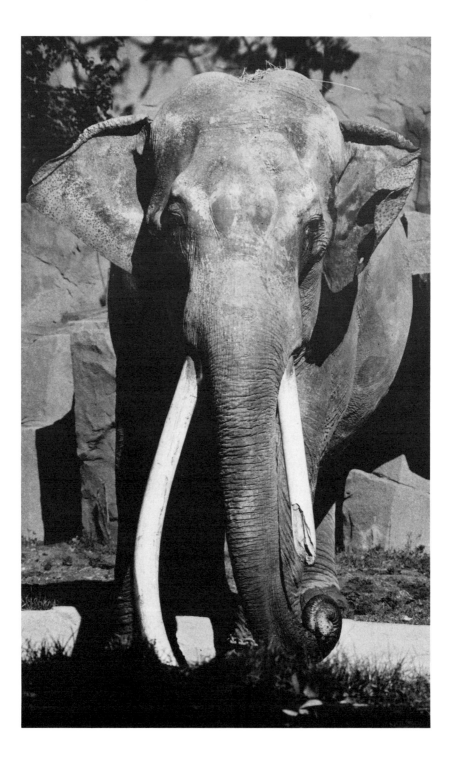

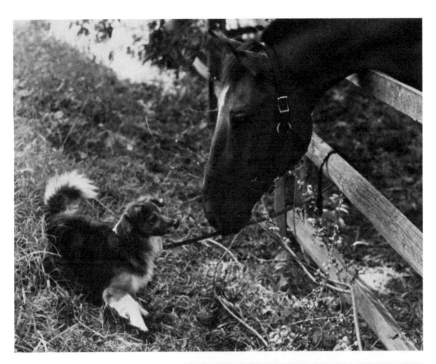

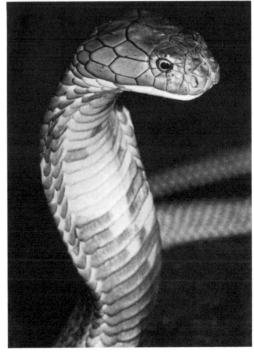

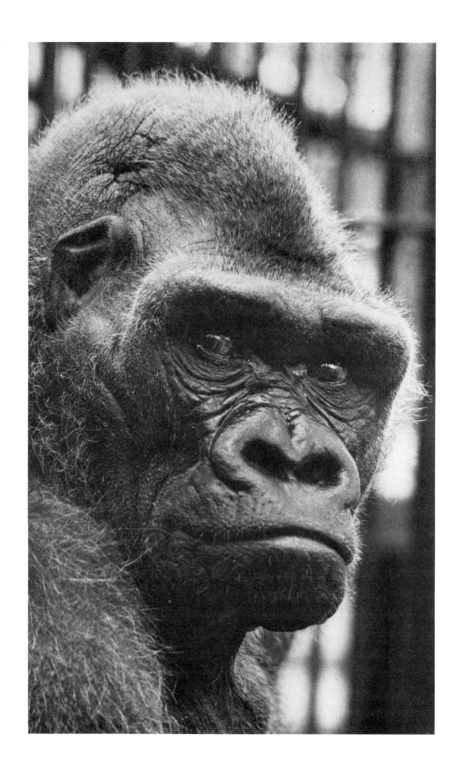

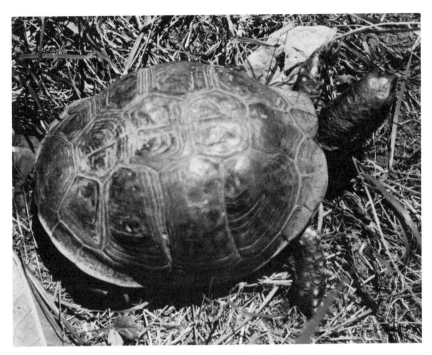

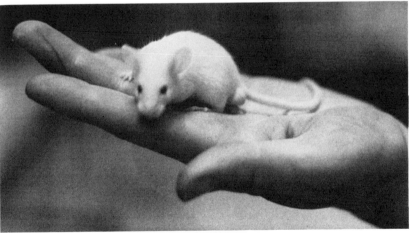

Top: The small box turtle is one of the longest-lived animals. Low metabolism helps explain its longevity.   *Barbara Ford*

Bottom: The high metabolism of this tiny white mouse helps explain its short life-span.   *Barbara Ford*

Opposite: Great apes have large brains, a characteristic that seems linked with long life. Massa, the world's oldest gorilla, was forty-nine in 1979.

Zoological Society of Philadelphia, Pennsylvania

work harder to produce the energy it needs. The body of a large mammal like the elephant, on the other hand, works much less hard to produce the needed energy. It has low metabolism. Cold-blooded animals such as reptiles and fish have low metabolism too, because they need less energy than warm-blooded animals. In general, the lower the metabolism, the longer the life-span.

Female animals tend to have slightly lower metabolism than males, which may help explain why females in most species live longer than males. But the different behavior of males and females probably has something to do with longevity too.

There are some puzzles about metabolism, however. Bats have a high metabolism, but some bats are believed to live over thirty years, far longer than other mammals their size. And birds have a higher metabolism, but they live much longer than small mammals.

George Sacher thinks birds may live a long time because they have a higher temperature than mammals. One of his formulas shows that when two animals have the same metabolic rate, the species with the higher temperature is likely to have a longer life. He also speculates that bats achieve a longer life in still another way. Insect-eating bats in temperate climates spend about 80 percent of their life in hibernation. During this state, they reduce their metabolism tenfold. So bats really use no more energy in their lifetime than small mammals that do not hibernate and die much sooner.

ANIMAL AND HUMAN
AGING

A housefly attached to a bent reed beats its wings rapidly. Just in back of the fly is a boxlike instrument with a light source called a "stroboscope." The stroboscope makes it possible to tell the speed of the fly's wingbeat. Dr. Morris Rockstein, a professor of physiology at the University of Miami School of Medicine, Coral Gables, Florida, has discovered that the speed of the wings of young flies is very fast, perhaps 8900 beats per minute. When flies grow older, the rate of their wingbeats drops sharply.

Rockstein is one of a number of scientists who are studying animal aging to learn more about human aging. Invertebrates, rats, mice, rabbits, carnivores, and primates are all being used by scientists as models for man in aging studies. Except for invertebrates like the fly, all the animals being studied are mammals, members of the same group we belong to. Many of their body parts have a structure similar to ours, and their bodies work in much the same ways as ours do.

But how can flies and other invertebrates serve as models for people when they are so different?

Surprisingly, invertebrates, too, have similarities to human beings. Some insects have cells, the smallest unit of life, that resemble ours, and insect and human bodies perform alike in

47

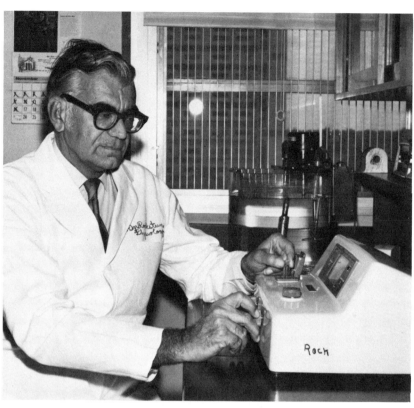

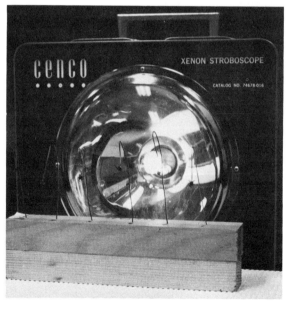

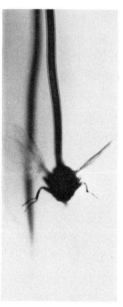

some ways. One researcher has discovered, for example, that the biochemistry of the insect flight muscle is similar to that of our liver and heart muscle. Insects also have other advantages as research subjects. They are small, they are available in large numbers, and they have a short life-span. A researcher can study many, many generations of a creature that lives only a month or so.

In some of his recent studies, Morris Rockstein has concentrated on flight and the flight muscle. He finds that among male and female houseflies, the animals fly many hours a day in their first few days of life but that the amount of flying drops off dramatically as they age. At the same time, the amount of an energy-producing substance, or enzyme, in the flight muscle decreases too. The flight muscle itself, however, doesn't seem to change.

As the male fly ages, he quickly loses most of his wings. Oddly enough, females keep their wings much longer. They also live twice as long as males.

Insects will be more widely used in aging research in the future, but the most popular animal model today is the rodent. One particular rat, the Fischer 344 inbred white rat, is used more than any other animal in aging studies. Over forty years ago, Dr. Clive M. McCay of Cornell University in Ithaca, New York, fed newly weaned rats about six weeks old a low-calorie diet. The underfed rats grew much more slowly than rats fed a normal diet. After keeping his rats on a low-calorie diet for various periods, McCay fed them normally again. The

Top: Morris Rockstein analyzes sample of housefly flight muscle.
Bottom left: The stroboscope measures the rapid wingbeat of flies attached to a bent reed in front of a light source.
Bottom right: A close-up of a fly in front of the stroboscope.
Overleaf: These four photographs show how a male housefly's wings change with age.   *Morris Rockstein*

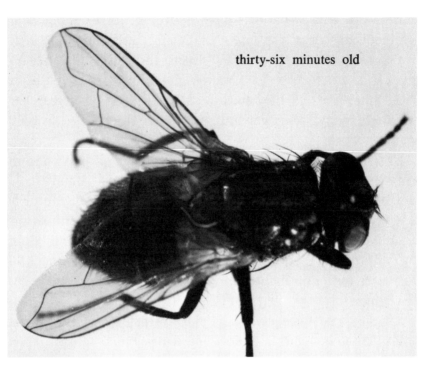

thirty-six minutes old

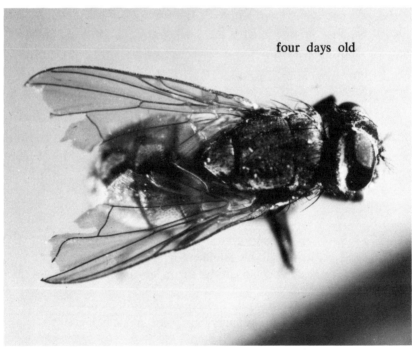

four days old

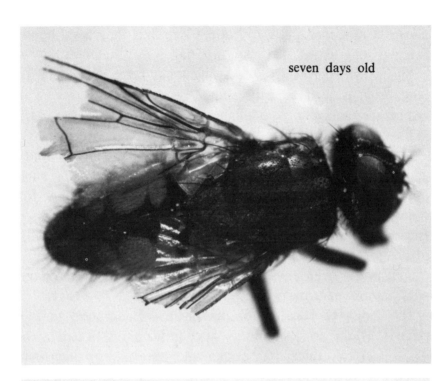

seven days old

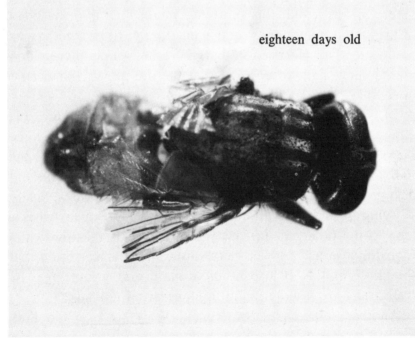

eighteen days old

underfed rats soon grew to normal size, but they lived about twice as long as rats fed a normal diet.

Since then, the McCay experiment has been repeated with other rats as well as with animals of various species. The results are the same. Something about a low-calorie diet early in life makes animals live longer.

One of the modern scientists who is using rodents to study aging is Professor Richard Dapson, the developer of the lens-protein method of aging mammals. His research animal for some of these studies is the wild old-field mouse. Professor Dapson found that old-field mice caught in an environment with plenty to eat showed fewer signs of age than old-field mice caught in a barren environment. He believes the stress of the poor environment makes mice age faster.

Dr. David E. Harrison of the Jackson Laboratory in Bar Harbor, Maine, uses laboratory mice in his aging research. He has joined two mice, one young and one old, so that their blood can intermingle. If something in the blood of the old mouse makes it old, this substance might flow into the blood of the young mouse and age it prematurely. In preliminary experiments, Dr. Harrison found that the young mouse does indeed show signs of age and that the old mouse shows signs of youth.

Dr. George A. Sacher of the Argonne Laboratory uses two different rodents in some of his aging studies. They look alike, but one, the house mouse, lives about three years at best, while the other, the white-footed mouse (a close relative of the old-field mouse), has a maximum age of about eight years. Sacher is trying to find out why one mouse lives more than twice as long as the other. So far, his research reveals that the white-footed mouse has a lower metabolism and a bigger brain than the house mouse. It also becomes mature at a later age. All these traits are usually found in longer-lived animals.

Another researcher, Dr. Ronald W. Hart of Ohio State University, has discovered that cell damage in the white-footed mouse is repaired more quickly than in the house mouse. This discovery is significant because it supports a theory of aging held by a number of scientists, including Sacher. According to this theory, aging is caused by damage to the body's cells from various causes. The body keeps making repairs on such damage throughout life, but eventually there is simply too much and the animal dies. The fact that damage in the body cells of the long-lived white-footed mouse is repaired more quickly than in the short-lived house mouse seems to show that aging is somehow connected with the efficiency of the repair mechanism within the body.

Other research by Dr. Hart and Dr. Richard B. Setlow of Brookhaven National Laboratory in Upton, New York, supports the damage theory. Hart and Setlow used invisible ultraviolet irradiation from a special lamp to damage cell cultures from seven different animals, ranging from the shrew to the human being. The animals that lived the longest, they report, are those in which damage caused by irradiation is repaired most quickly. Which animal cells are repaired the fastest of all? Human cells. The study shows that human cell damage is repaired about twice as efficiently as chimpanzee cell damage, and people live about twice as long.

According to Sacher, the research on irradiation damage suggests human beings may be able to lengthen their life-span in the future. Experts on ancient man tell us we began to change, or evolve, from an ape man into the creature we are today millions of years ago. During the last two million years, we increased our brain size about three times. Sacher believes that we increased our life-span from that of an ape to that of a human being at the same time we increased our brain size.

Two million years sounds like a long time, but in terms of evolution it is not. The fact that we changed so much in such a short time, argues Sacher, indicates the changes may depend on just a few genes, the basic unit of inheritance. If so, human beings may be able someday to become even more intelligent,

53

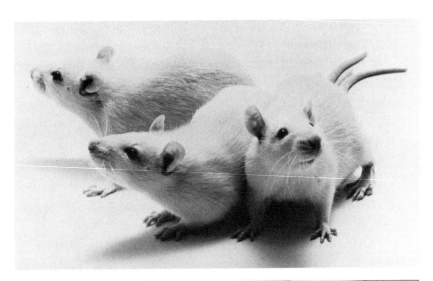

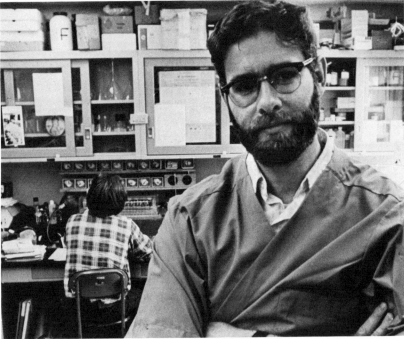

Top: These Fischer 344 inbred white rats, the most popular animal for aging studies, are raised in large numbers at the Charles River Breeding Laboratories, Wilmington, Massachusetts. *Charles River Breeding Laboratories*
Bottom: David E. Harrison   *Jackson Laboratory, Bar Harbor, Maine*
Opposite: Ronald W. Hart   *Ohio State University*

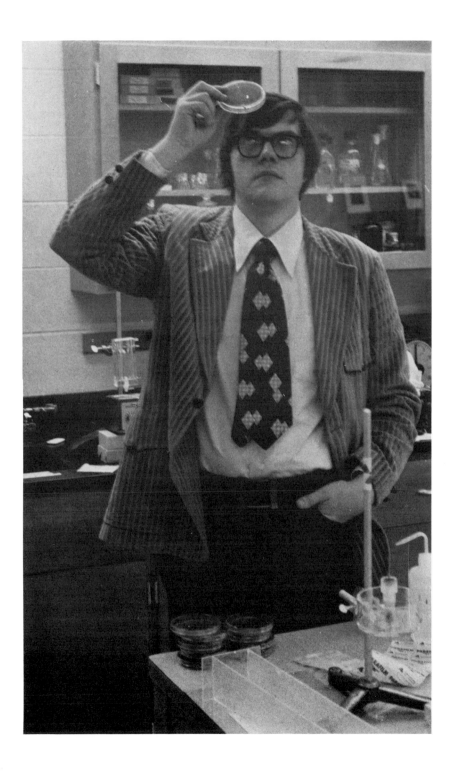

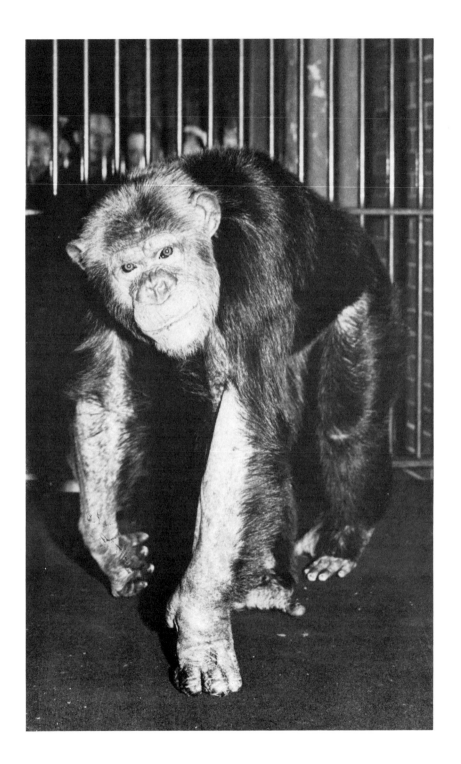

as well as longer-lived. If these changes are left to nature, they would take millions of years more, but people may be able to accomplish them in a much shorter time by modifying the genes.

The other theory of aging is that it is caused by a gene that programs the animal for death at a certain time. Each species has its own aging program. There is animal research to support this theory, too. Some years ago Dr. Leonard Hayflick of Stanford University discovered that cultures of the cells of various animals reproduce themselves, or double, a certain number of times before they die. Cells from children reproduce about fifty times before they die out, cells from old human beings about thirty to forty times. House mouse cells reproduce only about twelve times, but cells of the longer-lived white-footed mouse reproduce about twenty times. Chicken cells reproduce about twenty-five times. Many scientists have repeated this experiment with the same results.

Which theory of aging will turn out to be the correct one? Or will some new theory win acceptance? Whatever happens, research on animal life-spans is bound to play an important part in unraveling the mystery of aging.

Heinie lived at the Lincoln Park Zoo for forty-seven years, a record for male chimpanzees. New research shows that chimpanzees repair damage to their cells only half as efficiently as human beings.
Lincoln Park Zoological Gardens, Chicago, Illinois

APPENDIX
MAXIMUM LONGEVITIES

*achieved in the wild

INVERTEBRATES

quahog clam	149 years*
Arctica islandica	
sea anemone	80–90 years
Cerus pedenunculatus	
human tapeworm	35 years
Dibothriocephalus latens	
queen termite	25 years*
Neotermes castaneus	
17-year cicada	
(as immature grub)	17 years*
(as adult)	5 weeks*
Magicicada septendecim	
queen ant	15 years
Formica fusca	
worker ant	7 years
Formica fusca	
queen honey bee	6 years
Apis mellifera	
earthworm	6 years
Lumbricus terrestris	
worker honey bee	6 months
Apis mellifera	
housefly (female)	67 days
Musca domestica	
housefly (male)	59 days
Musca domestica	

58

mayfly	1 day*
Ephemeroptera order	

black Seychelles tortoise	152 years
Testudo sumeirei	
Carolina, or eastern, box turtle	129 years*
Terrapene carolina	
Galapagos tortoise	over 100 years
Testudo elephantopus	
tuatara	77 years
Sphenodon punctatus	
snapping turtle	62 years
Macrochelys temmincki	
red-ear turtle	over 60 years
Chrysemys scripta elegans	
American alligator	56 years
Alligator mississippiensis	
North American musk turtle	52 years
Sternotherus odoratus	
boa constrictor	40 years
Constrictor constrictor	
common toad	36 years
Bufo bufo	
cottonmouth water moccasin	21 years
Agkistrodon piscivorus	
bullfrog	16 years
Rana catesbeiana	
garter snake	10 years
Thamnophis sirtalis	
anole lizard	4 years
Anolis carolinensis	

sturgeon	82 years*
Acipenser transmontanus	
European catfish, or wels	60 years*
Silurus glanis	
American eel	50 years
Anguilla rostrada	
freshwater carp	47 years
Cyprinus carpio	
goldfish	40 years
Carassius auratus	

59

Australian school shark	32 years*
Galeorhinus australis	
longnose gar	30 years
Lepisosteus osseus	
striped bass	24 years
Roccus saxatilis	
Atlantic herring	19 years
Clupea harengus	
walleyed pike	18 years
Stizostedion vitreum	
Atlantic salmon	13 years
Salmo salar	
Pacific salmon (sockeye)	7 years*
Oncorhynchus nerka	
guppy	6 years
Lebistes reticulatus	
goby	1 year
Gobiidae family	

BIRDS

eagle owl	68 years
Bubo bubo	
Andean condor	65 years
Vultur gryphus	
Asiatic crane	60 years
Grus leucogeranus	
greater sulphur-crested cockatoo	56 years
Kakatoe galerita	
white pelican	51 years
Pelecanus onocrotalus	
African gray parrot	50 years
Psittacus erithacus	
golden eagle	46 years
Aquila chrysaetos	
blue and yellow macaw	43 years
Ara ararauna	
herring gull	41 years; 31 years*
Larus argentatus	
emperor penguin	34 years
Aptenodytes forsteri	
domestic pigeon	30 years
Columba livia	
English sparrow	23 years
Passer domesticus	

canary	22 years
Serinus canarius	
Indian hill mynah	20 years
Gracula religiosa	
budgerigar, or "budgie"	15 years
Melopsittacus undulatus	
blue jay	14 years*
Cyanocitta cristata	
mockingbird	12 years*
Mimus polyglottos	
domestic chicken	10 years
Gallus gallus	
black-capped chickadee	10 years*
Parus atricapillus	

MAMMALS

Indian elephant	69–77 years
Elephas maximus	
sperm whale	77 years*
Physeter catodon	
orangutan	59 years
Pongo pygmaeus abelii	
pilot whale	50 years*
Globicephala melaena	
spiny anteater, or echidna	49 years
Tachyglossus aculeatus	
gorilla	49 years
Gorilla gorilla	
chimpanzee	49 years
Chimpansee troglodytes	
white-faced capuchin monkey	49 years
Cebus capucinus	
domestic horse	46 years
Equus caballus	
hippopotamus	43 years*
Hippopotamus amphibius	
black bear	41 years*
Ursus americanus	
African black rhinoceros	40 years
Diceros bicornis	
bottle-nosed dolphin	35 years*
Tursiops truncatus	
polar bear	34 years
Thalarctos maritimus	

Indian fruit bat *Pteropus giganteus*	31	years
domestic cat *Felis catus*	31	years
lion *Leo leo*	30	years
domestic dog *Canis familiaris*	27	years
tiger (Bengal) *Leo tigris*	26	years
gray squirrel *Sciurus carolinensis*	23	years
leopard *Leo pardus*	23	years
coyote *Canis latrans*	21	years
domestic cow *Bos taurus*	over 20	years
white-tailed deer *Odocoileus virginianus*	20	years
timber wolf *Canis lupus*	19	years
red fox *Vulpes fulva*	12	years
guinea pig, or cavy *Cavia porcellus*	8	years
chipmunk *Tamias striatus*	8	years
Norway rat *Rattus norvegicus*	6	years
gerbil *Gerbillus gerbillus*	5	years
golden hamster *Mesocricetus auratus*	3	years
house mouse *Mus musculus*	3	years
shrew (common) *Sorex araneus*	18	months*

INDEX

* indicates illustration

63